Contents

Acknowledgements   *page 4*

Foreword by Angela Greatley   *page 5*

Glossary of terms   *page 6*

Chapter 1   **Why we need intermediate care**   *page 9*
Introduction   *page 9*
The extent of the problem   *page 10*
User vignettes   *page 10*
The problem of somatisation   *page 11*
The policy background   *page 12*

Chapter 2   **The Intermediate Care Model**   *page 15*
The model and how it works   *page 15*
What does the team do?   *page 16*
Expected outcomes   *page 17*

Chapter 3   **The need for intermediate care – a case study**   *page 19*
The Intermediate Care Collaborative Project   *page 19*
The Primary Care Intermediate Mental Health Service (PIMHS) in
Ipswich   *page 19*

Chapter 4   **Setting up an intermediate care team**   *page 23*
Introduction   *page 23*
Preparation   *page 23*
Implementation   *page 25*
The intermediate care team in practice   *page 29*

Chapter 5   **Assessing the need for intermediate care in your locality**   *page 33*
Introduction   *page 33*
The prevalence of mental illness in a locality   *page 34*
The need for intermediate care   *page 37*

Chapter 6   **Evaluating intermediate care**   *page 43*
Introduction   *page 43*
Evaluating intermediate care   *page 43*
Analysis   *page 45*
Ethics and local research governance   *page 46*

References and further reading   *page 47*

Acknowledgements

We would like to thank staff at the following primary care trusts (PCTs) who are participating in the Intermediate Care Collaborative project:

East Lincolnshire
Barking & Dagenham
Ipswich
North, South and Central Liverpool
Southampton
Waltham Forest
Wakefield West and Eastern Wakefield

In particular we would like to thank the following contributing authors:

Graham Durcan, Deputy Director Service Development & Criminal Justice and Mental Health Programme Lead, The Sainsbury Centre for Mental Health
Dr Shahid Dadabhoy, GP, Chingford, London and Professional Executive Committee Mental Health Lead, Waltham Forest PCT

We would also like to thank:

Addah Nyawo
Mary Roberts
Roy Marsh
Karen Guinness
Gillian Garden
Maisie Allen
Bernard Hannah
Christa Drennan
Tony Ranzetta

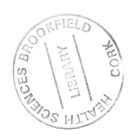

The Neglected Majority
Developing intermediate mental health care in primary care

John Hague
GP and Mental Health Lead, Ipswich
Independent consultant to Primary Care, The Sainsbury Centre for Mental Health

Alan Cohen
Director of Primary Care
The Sainsbury Centre for Mental Health

ISBN: 1 870480 66 X

Published by
The Sainsbury Centre for Mental Health
134-138 Borough High Street
London SE1 1LB
Tel: 020 7827 8300
Fax: 020 7403 9482
www.scmh.org.uk

The Sainsbury Centre for Mental Health (SCMH) is a charity that works to improve the quality of life for people with severe mental health problems. It carries out research, development and training work to influence policy and practice in health and social care. SCMH was founded in 1985 by the Gatsby Charitable Foundation, one of the Sainsbury Family Charitable Trusts, from which it receives core funding. SCMH is affiliated to the Institute of Psychiatry at King's College, London.

A charitable company limited by guarantee registered in England and Wales no. 4373019
Charity registration no. 1091 1156

Design: www.intertype.com
Printing: Nuffield Press, UK

Foreword

This publication is intended to offer a new way of supporting a group of people whose needs are often not catered for within current mental health service provision. This 'neglected majority' has common and enduring mental health problems, such as depression and anxiety, and requires greater support than primary care can provide on its own, but does not qualify for specialist NHS mental health services.

Intermediate care may be able to fill that gap in service provision, improving people's lives through not only mental health care, but support with other issues such as housing, employment, benefits or relationships. This focus on the wider needs of the individual can help to keep people in their homes and jobs and support them to live the lives they want.

Intermediate care has been pioneered by the Sainsbury Centre for Mental Health (SCMH) through its work with the Intermediate Care Collaborative Project, run in sites across the country. The teams which have been set up through this scheme have already begun to make a difference to people's lives and will hopefully be the first of many. This publication draws on the experiences of these teams to provide practical step-by-step guidance to setting up a successful intermediate care team.

Intermediate care is an innovative new approach to supporting a 'neglected majority'. By harnessing the experience of pilot projects such as those set up by the Intermediate Care Collaborative, it takes us beyond national prescriptions and towards a service which caters for the holistic needs of every person.

I hope this guide will inspire others to take up the challenge of providing a better service for this group of people as part of the continued modernisation of mental health care.

Angela Greatley
Chief Executive
The Sainsbury Centre for Mental Health

Glossary of terms

Evidence-based intervention
A treatment which has research evidence supporting its effectiveness published in the scientific literature.

Expert by Experience
(Often lay) people who have had a mental health condition and work to improve the experience of others using services. See also 'expert patient'.

Expert Patient
An expert by experience who has undergone a specific training course to become an 'expert patient'.

Gateway Worker
A qualified, experienced, mental health professional, who may come from a nursing, psychology, occupational therapy, counselling, or social work background, and work as a community psychiatric nurse or primary care mental health worker (PCMHW). They have a specific role in being a link worker between primary and secondary care. One of the targets in the *National Service Framework for Mental Health* (DH, 1999) was the establishment of 500 gateway workers nationally.

Practitioner with special interest (PwSI)
A doctor (GPwSI) or nurse who works mostly in primary care, but has a special interest in a particular field, and is employed as a 'sub specialist' to provide a service in this field. In this publication the special interest referred to is mental health.

Graduate primary care mental health worker
A recent graduate (usually of psychology), in a specific junior training post in primary care mental health, often with no previous clinical experience, and initially requiring supervision in their work.

Guided Bibliotherapy
A form of therapy in which the patient works through a structured book as a means of treating their condition. The work is 'guided' by brief consultations with a health care worker.

Mental Health Lead
A GP who is employed by a PCT to advise on mental health issues.

Primary Care Mental Health Worker (PCMHW)
A qualified, experienced, mental health professional, who may come from a nursing, psychology, occupational therapy, counselling, or social work background. They are able to work unsupervised, and be responsible for and manage a caseload. They have often previously worked as part of a CMHT, but will need to have extra skills to work in primary care. These workers could be gateway workers, but have a potentially wider job description.

Rating Scale
A brief questionnaire, usually completed by a client and scored by a health professional, that allows standardised assessment and monitoring of a client's mental state. Examples include the Hospital Anxiety and Depression Scale (HADS) and the Depression, Anxiety and Stress Scale (DASS).

Read Code
A coding system for recording diagnoses and treatment in UK primary care IT systems.

Reattribution

A treatment method which enables patients to understand how the basis of their symptoms is psychological rather than physical.

Somatisation

A disorder in which people present frequently to the doctor with recurrent and frequently changing physical symptoms that cannot be medically explained.

Triage

A process undertaken at initial interview (sometimes on the telephone), where an experienced practitioner arrives at a working diagnosis, and decides on the likely broad category of intervention that will be needed for a client.

Abbreviations

A&E	Accident and Emergency
CAB	Citizens Advice Bureau
CBT	Cognitive Behavioural Therapy
CMHT	Community Mental Health Team
GP	General Practitioner
GPwSI	General Practitioner with a Special Interest (in mental health)
LIT	Local Implementation Team for the National Service Framework for Mental Health
nGMS	The 2004 GP contract between the Department of Health and GPs
NSF-MH	National Service Framework for Mental Health
PHCT	Primary Health Care Team
PCMHW	Primary Care Mental Health Worker
PCT	Primary Care Trust
PCT PEC	PCT Professional Executive Committee
PCT Board	PCT Board of Directors
PwSI	Practitioner with a Special Interest (in mental health)

Box 1: The Intermediate Care Model

A team is developed within a locality that provides care for people who have common mental health problems which cannot be managed in confidence in primary care, but who are inappropriate for specialist mental health services, and who:

■ Have had two evidence-based interventions, such as CBT or a course of medication for that mental health condition and are still symptomatic, OR

■ Have had at least one evidence-based intervention for that condition AND their housing or employment is at risk because of that mental health condition, OR

■ Have had at least one evidence-based intervention for that mental health condition AND their co-existing physical health disorder is exacerbated by the mental health condition.

The team is usually the same size as the community mental health team (CMHT) in the locality, and it serves the same population as the CMHT. The membership of the team can reflect local need, and local resources, but in general it will draw on the human resources and personnel that are already working on mental health issues in the community. Membership of the team includes: health professionals providing a variety of talking therapies within primary care services; professionals from the local authority who provide expertise on housing, benefit and employment matters; and voluntary sector representatives providing access to further talking therapies. The team also includes users and carers providing telephone follow-up and support to current users of the team.

The team will provide evidence-based interventions in line with NICE guidance (NICE, 2004a, 2004b) for people who fit the criteria described above.

CHAPTER 1

Why we need intermediate care

Introduction

At present, 30% of primary care consultations have a mental health component (SCMH, 2002). The World Health Organisation forecasts that depression will be the most common chronic health problem globally by 2010 (Murray & Lopez, 1996). In the UK an estimated four million people experience mental health problems, the majority of them depression and anxiety (Layard, 2005).

Since the early 1990s government policy has prioritised the care of people suffering from severe mental illnesses such as bipolar disorder (manic depression) and schizophrenia. This was reinforced by the *National Service Framework for Mental Health* (NSF-MH) and its early implementation (DH, 1999). The result is that secondary care focuses on the care of people with severe mental illness and primary care supports a large group of people with common mental health problems, such as anxiety and depression. It is estimated in *The National Service Framework for Mental Health* that 91% of people with a mental health problem are now cared for entirely within primary care (DH, 1999).

Common and enduring mental health problems

Of this 91%, there is a group of people who have common and enduring mental health problems and who do not respond to the treatment offered by their GP. These people often have complex socio-economic needs relating to housing, employment, benefits, or relationship issues. These problems may also affect the health of their carers. Unless these needs are addressed recovery may not take place. Refugees and asylum seekers with mental health problems in particular may have complex needs, which may be compounded by communication problems if they do not speak English well, and the severity of the past trauma that caused them to become refugees or asylum seekers.

Historically, people in this group have been referred to specialist mental health services by their GPs, assessed in a process that can take two workers up to two hours, and then told that they do not meet the criteria for acceptance. At this point the patient has nowhere to go, feeling that they have been rejected by both primary and secondary care. The GP is frustrated by the inability of the system to help their patient, and the community mental health team (CMHT) is frustrated by the 'inappropriate referral'. The time and resources tied up in these 'inappropriate assessments' could be better used in providing a service that actually addresses the person's needs, enabling secondary care to focus on people who have severe mental conditions and primary care to support people with less severe problems.

Intermediate care

Intermediate care provides a solution to these difficulties. This innovative way of working is based in primary care but brings together a group of workers who are already employed locally in the health, social care, local authority and voluntary sectors. Team membership (depending on local circumstances) might include people from primary care, social care, housing, employment, expert patient and counselling backgrounds. The aim is to support patients in all aspects of their lives. Typically, the team might provide therapies such as cognitive behavioural therapy (CBT), group work and support in developing problem solving skills. They might also help the user to obtain advice about practical issues such as housing, benefits and employment.

The Intermediate Care Collaborative Project

The Sainsbury Centre for Mental Health is collaborating with a number of primary care trusts (PCTs) around the country to develop intermediate care. This publication pulls together the early experiences of this work and provides a simple and practical guide to setting up an intermediate care team. Much of the experience of intermediate care services referenced in the publication comes from the Primary Care Intermediate Mental Health Service (PIMHS) in Ipswich. For further details on the project as a whole and on the PIMHS service, see Chapter 3.

Based on the experience of the Intermediate Care Collaborative Project, this publication shows how to assess the need for such a service in your area or primary care practice with step-by-step guides on planning the service and setting up the team. Finally, it looks at the crucial aspect of evaluating the impact of the service.

This publication is aimed at all those who are interested in developing services for people with common and enduring mental health problems. It will be of interest to people working in primary and secondary care, social care, housing, employment and the voluntary sector. It will be of particular interest to mental health commissioners, members of PCT boards and Local Implementation Teams for the *National Service Framework for Mental Health*.

The extent of the problem

There have been few studies that have focused specifically on people who have common and enduring mental health problems with complex needs, so it is difficult to assess the number of people in this group. However, some inferences can be drawn from national and international data, and from studies associated with the practical experience of the intermediate care teams set up through the Intermediate Care Collaborative Project.

For example, figures from the NICE Depression Guidelines (NICE, 2004a) show that 20% of individuals with depression are still unwell two years after diagnosis. Figures from the USA suggest that with usual primary care this number is closer to 59% (Rost *et al.*, 2002). Truly this is a 'neglected majority'.

If the needs of a person with mental health problems are not catered for by either primary or secondary care, it is likely that they will suffer in other areas of their lives, particularly whether they are able to work. Many are therefore out of work and receive Incapacity Benefit. About one million people are out of work due to mental illness and receive Incapacity Benefit – more than there are unemployed people on Jobseekers' Allowance (Layard, 2004). But less than 10% of these people are in contact with specialist mental health services (Social Exclusion Unit, 2004). An audit of one practice's referrals to intermediate care in Ipswich (Hague, 2005) identified a very high proportion of those in contact with the service who were not employed or were frequently absent from work. The figures were considerably higher than the average among people with mental health conditions (SCMH, 2003).

User vignettes

These fictional vignettes illustrate the sort of problems seen in intermediate care, and the breadth of interventions and techniques that can be employed.

■ Robin is a 48 year old man, who has become unemployed. He develops depression, responding well at first to treatment from his GP. When he is well enough to look for work he relapses. He discloses that he has a specific learning difficulty and finds the 'usual' help at the Job Centre very hard to access. He finally goes onto Incapacity Benefit, but then has it withdrawn. In intermediate care (to which he is referred by Job Centre Plus) Robin has several sessions of CBT, and is helped back into the workplace by being introduced to the local volunteer centre. Some weeks later he is accompanied by an advice worker to an appointment with Job Centre Plus.

■ Sarah is a 55 year old woman with longstanding depression, who has previously been discharged from the CMHT. She lost her job last year, and is sleeping on a friend's sofa. She also suffers from a chronic chest complaint. She was seen for assessment by the intermediate care team primary care mental health worker (PCMHW), and then seen by a graduate primary care mental health worker three times to address her benefit and accommodation issues. Following that she saw a PCMHW four times for CBT work to address anxiety and depression, using guided bibliotherapy as 'homework'. By the end of treatment she is beginning to look at volunteering.

■ Stephen is a 37 year old man with anxiety and depression. He is suffering from his second episode of depression in two years. He is not responding to medication prescribed by his GP. The illness is affecting family life; he is just managing to work part time, but the lack of money coming in to the family is a problem. He is seen for assessment by the intermediate care team and five follow-ups plus several phone calls. CBT-based work concentrates on anxiety and panic and on understanding depression. Assertiveness issues became more apparent, so this area is concentrated on in the last three sessions, along with computer based guided bibliotherapy. He is able to utilise all techniques to good effect and his mood settles after his medication is optimised by the team's GP with a special interest (GPwSI), and other medical conditions are excluded. By the end of treatment he is looking for full time work.

The problem of somatisation

There is also a group of people who come to their GP with physical symptoms but no detectable physical condition. They are frequent attenders in primary care and are often referred to hospital for investigations, yet infrequently have the psychological problems behind their presentation addressed. This is often very frustrating for the patient and consumes a lot of NHS resources.

Box 2: Somatisation

- 20-50% of district general hospital patients have psychiatric problems, less than half of which are recognised (Bass, 2003).

- Less than 1 in 10 of these are referred to mental health services (Bolton, 2003).

- One third of all medical outpatients have medically unexplained symptoms, rising to 50% for outpatients in cardiology, gastroenterology and neurology (Bass, 2003).

- One American study showed that the mean cost per patient per year of patients with medically unexplained symptoms is £1,040. Most of this cost is unnecessary admission and investigation (Barsky et al., 2001)

- A study in the UK estimated that each 'somatising patient' costs £955 in secondary care (Reid et al., 2002).

- 20% of male inpatients have alcohol related problems (Bolton, 2003).

- Up to 5% of patients attending A&E have psychiatric problems as the main reason for attendance (Bolton, 2003).

Practitioners in primary and intermediate care are uniquely placed to help this group; those working in hospitals are less likely to be in possession of the patient's complete details (although this should change with the introduction of national electronic health records).

Recent advice from the USA (Abbas, 2005) suggests that somatisation should become a diagnosis that is not reached by exclusion of physical problems, but should be suspected at the outset if a patient seems obviously anxious. Conducting an 'emotion focused interview' will then help to rule somatisation in or out. If this is identified, the patient may be helped to understand how the basis of their symptoms is psychological rather than physical through a process of 'reattribution'. An excellent patient resource which can be helpful for this group of patients can be downloaded from: www.mentalneurologicalprimaryc are.org/downloads/primary_care/10_unexplained_physical_complaints.pdf.

In Chapter 5 there are several audit tools to identify how many people may have this condition in a particular practice or area.

The policy background

Supporting People with Long Term Conditions (2005)

Intermediate care is supported by current Department of Health policies on the care of people with long term conditions. Figure 1 shows the 'pyramid of care' developed by US health provider Kaiser Permanente which divides the population of patients with long term conditions into three distinct groups based on their degree of need. This figure was reproduced in the Department of Health policy document *Supporting People with Long Term Conditions* (DH, 2005).

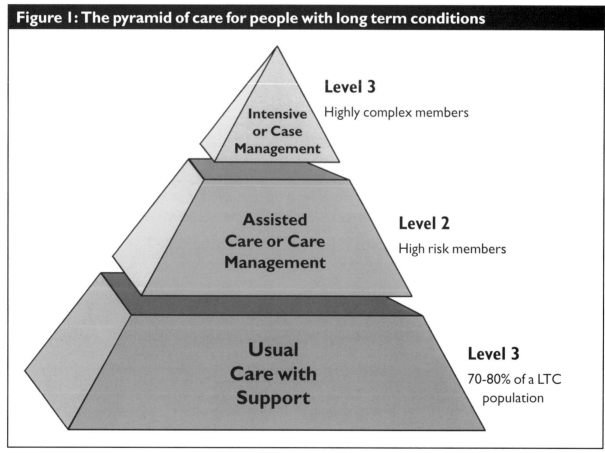

Figure 1: The pyramid of care for people with long term conditions

Level 3
Intensive or Case Management
Highly complex members

Level 2
Assisted Care or Care Management
High risk members

Level 3
Usual Care with Support
70-80% of a LTC population

LTC = long term condition

The intention is that different levels of risk or severity of illness receive different types of intervention. For diabetes and coronary heart disease this is an obvious, and already implemented, process. Not everybody with angina is immediately offered coronary artery bypass graft. Not everybody with diabetes is immediately started on insulin.

For severe and enduring mental illness (schizophrenia and bipolar disorder) it could be argued that the structure of mental health teams reflect this approach already, with CMHTs providing a less intensive form of support compared to assertive outreach teams, who provide care to people with very severe and disorganised problems. The applicability of this model to common mental health conditions was focused on in the NICE Depression Guidelines (NICE, 2004a), examined later in this chapter.

National Service Framework for Mental Health (1999)

The *National Service Framework for Mental Health* (NSF-MH), published in 1999, made clear that the first priority of specialist mental health teams was those with a severe and enduring mental illness. The definition provided is predominantly people with a psychotic illness. One of the unexpected consequences of this very clear separation between the role of primary and secondary care services was that in many areas the service offered by mental health trusts is different to that required by the referring GPs. GPs not only require a referral and treatment service for people with a severe and enduring mental illness, but also require an advice and assessment service for people who have 'common' mental health problems. This mismatch results in complaints from both sides about unrealistic expectations, failure to be responsive, and the oft-quoted 'inappropriate referrals'.

NHS Plan (2000)

The *NHS Plan* (DH, 2000) described the creation of new posts called graduate primary care mental health workers. Again, the principle of such a post was welcomed, but concerns were expressed about the implementation (SCMH, 2002). There was considerable fear that these relatively young and inexperienced professionals would be left unsupported in the community trying to help people with complex mental health problems which experienced GPs could not manage with confidence. Several PCTs around the country have experimented with some success at setting up different types of team to look at how these workers could be incorporated into either primary care or specialist services.

Social Exclusion Unit Report (2004)

The Social Exclusion Unit report published in 2004 looked at the consequences of mental health problems particularly on employment opportunities (Social Exclusion Unit, 2004). One of the most important aspects of this publication was that it did not limit its analysis to people in contact with mental health trusts, which by definition would continue to give priority to people with severe and enduring mental illness. The consequence was that it became clear that there were many people with a common condition who also had problems with employment or housing, yet were inappropriate for care by specialist mental health services.

NICE Guidelines (2004)

In December 2004, the National Institute for Health and Clinical Excellence (NICE) published guidelines for the management of depression (NICE, 2004a) and for the management of generalised anxiety disorder and panic disorder (NICE, 2004b). The guidelines were welcomed as they provide a rigorous evidence base for providing care for a group of disorders that are both common and cause significant distress and disability.

The guidelines have provided an opportunity to focus attention on a group of people whose care is not necessarily the responsibility of specialist mental health teams, yet for whom primary care sometimes struggles to provide all the different aspects of care which will benefit them.

The guidelines on depression also highlighted the concept of 'stepped care' (Figure 2), which is related to the Kaiser Permanente 'pyramid of care' referenced in the Department of Health publication *Supporting People with Long Term Conditions* (Figure 1). The NICE depression guidelines suggest that this model should also be applied to the care of people with common mental health conditions.

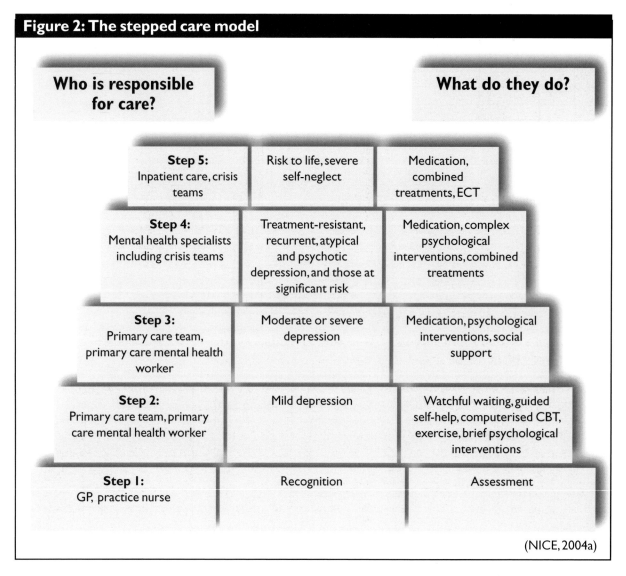

Figure 2: The stepped care model

Who is responsible for care?		What do they do?
Step 5: Inpatient care, crisis teams	Risk to life, severe self-neglect	Medication, combined treatments, ECT
Step 4: Mental health specialists including crisis teams	Treatment-resistant, recurrent, atypical and psychotic depression, and those at significant risk	Medication, complex psychological interventions, combined treatments
Step 3: Primary care team, primary care mental health worker	Moderate or severe depression	Medication, psychological interventions, social support
Step 2: Primary care team, primary care mental health worker	Mild depression	Watchful waiting, guided self-help, computerised CBT, exercise, brief psychological interventions
Step 1: GP, practice nurse	Recognition	Assessment

(NICE, 2004a)

All people with mental health problems access Step 1. Progression up the steps depends on need; people will only progress up the steps if there is a failure of response at the current step. Currently, mental health trusts provide care for steps 4 and 5, and primary care provides care covering steps 1 and 2. However, there is often a gap in current service provision at the Step 3 level.

The people who need care at Step 3 are those who have not responded to treatment provided by routine primary care, need more intensive support and treatment, including CBT, and frequently have co-existing physical health complaints, and/or social problems such as housing and unemployment – the client group for intermediate care.

CHAPTER 2

The Intermediate Care Model

The model and how it works

A team is developed within a locality that provides care for people who have common mental health problems which cannot be managed in confidence in primary care, but who are inappropriate for specialist mental health services, and who:

- Have had two evidence-based interventions, such as CBT or a course of medication for that mental health condition and are still symptomatic, OR

- Have had at least one evidence-based intervention for that condition AND their housing or employment is at risk because of that mental health condition, OR

- Have had at least one evidence-based intervention for that mental health condition AND their co-existing physical health disorder is exacerbated by the mental health condition.

The team is usually the same size as the community mental health team (CMHT) in the locality, and it serves the same population as the CMHT. The membership of the team can reflect local need, and local resources, but in general it will draw on the human resources and personnel that are already working on mental health issues in the community. In this way, the current workforce focuses more specifically on an 'at risk' group, whilst the staffing and membership of community mental health teams are not denuded to staff the new team.

Membership of the team includes: health professionals providing a variety of talking therapies within primary care services; professionals from the local authority who provide expertise on housing, benefit and employment matters; and voluntary sector representatives providing access to further talking therapies. The team also includes users and carers providing telephone follow-up and support to current users of the team.

The team will provide evidence-based interventions in line with NICE guidance (NICE, 2004a, 2004b) for people who fit the criteria described above.

Using the current workforce to provide a different, more targeted service lies at the heart of the Department of Health's modernisation agenda, as it uses the existing expertise in the most effective fashion. Since these personnel are already working in this area, and there are no new professional posts being created, the costs associated with setting up a new team are not excessive, although it would not be realistic to expect there to be no 'start up' costs.

What does the team do?

The following provides an outline of the work of an intermediate care team. Teams may provide some or all of these interventions for their clients:

- Brief therapy

- Cognitive behavioural therapy (CBT)

- Guided bibliotherapy/computerised CBT

- Problem solving

- Group work

- Advise GPs to optimise medication. (Only experienced workers such as PwSIs should do this.)

- Arrange appointments with partner organisations (actually arranging appointments, and even accompanying clients to other services is much more likely to be successful than simply providing clients with the telephone number and expecting them to take action) such as:
  - Housing
  - CAB (debt and legal issues)
  - Benefits advice
  - Job Centre Plus
  - Counselling
  - Volunteer bureau

- Review progress

- Telephone review, by qualified workers, graduate primary care mental health workers, volunteers, or experts by experience

- Change intervention if necessary.

After the intervention, the team has a number of options:

- Review

- Discharge if appropriate

- Change intervention

- Refer on to CMHT, or other part of secondary care.

Expected outcomes

There are a number of expected outcomes as a consequence of introducing an intermediate care service:

1. **Improved mental health**
    There will be a measured improvement in symptoms and signs of mental health disorders. This will be associated with more appropriate use of specialist mental health services.

2. **Improved physical health**
    There will be a measured improvement in symptoms and signs of long term physical health conditions. This will be associated with more appropriate use of acute health care services.

3. **Improved outcomes in employment opportunities**
    Users of the service will be able to access all the opportunities that are available so that they can make the best individual choice as to when, how, and what sort of rehabilitation will be most appropriate for their individual needs.

4. **Improved outcomes in accommodation**
    Users of the service will be able to access all the opportunities that are available so that they are able to make the best individual choice that will be most appropriate for their individual needs.

5. **Economic benefits**
    There will be some cost benefits associated with this team, but the immediately realisable savings may not come to the PCT, as savings associated with employment or housing will be experienced by the Exchequer and not at a local health level. Further details are available in the audit of the Ipswich intermediate care service by Tony Ranzetta (2005).

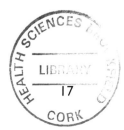

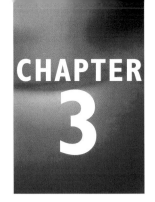

CHAPTER 3

The need for intermediate care – a case study

The Intermediate Care Collaborative Project

The Sainsbury Centre for Mental Health has collaborated with seven primary care trusts around the country to pilot this way of working.

Waltham Forest, and Barking and Dagenham PCT are scheduled to begin introducing a stepped care model in late 2005. Potential developments are ongoing in Liverpool, Southampton and Wakefield. East Lincolnshire PCT took part initially, but was then unable to participate, after making several key contributions. The pilot site in Ipswich, the Primary Care Intermediate Mental Health Service (PIMHS), has been operational since 31 January 2005.

The Primary Care Intermediate Mental Health Service (PIMHS) in Ipswich

The Primary Care Intermediate Mental Health Service (PIMHS) in Ipswich was the first operational intermediate mental health care team delivered as a result of the Sainsbury Centre for Mental Health Intermediate Care Collaborative.

PIMHS was set up in 2004-5 and began seeing patients living in Ipswich, on 31 January 2005. The team consists of a manager/mental health worker, two primary care mental health workers (registered mental health nurses), a secretary, a part time practitioner with a special interest in mental health (a psychiatrist, but could otherwise be a GPwSI) and an advice worker from East Suffolk Mind. It is supported by a network of agreements with local housing, advice, volunteer and employment services.

The need for intermediate care in Ipswich

A number of audits were undertaken by Ipswich PCT prior to setting up the team, showing how patients often 'revolved' from primary to secondary care, with their needs never being met.

- An audit in Ipswich general practices (Henshall, 2003) showed that an average of 1.35 patients per thousand per week had complex, enduring mental health problems, neither suitable for primary care, nor appropriate for referral to the secondary services. This is about 194 patients seen in practices every week in Ipswich.

- An audit of CMHT referrals in the town (Roberts, 2004) showed that of around 50 referrals received per month, 43% were returned to primary care with no treatment.

- The Acute Assessment (crisis resolution) Team in Ipswich (Little, 2003) averaged one 'inappropriate referral' per day from primary care – these were referred back to primary care with no other action being taken. Most admissions did not come from primary care, but were from specialist services.

The volume of referrals to the PIMHS team

In a typical PCT of 200,000 people there will be around 21,800 people who suffer from depression, anxiety, or other form of neuroses. A further 500 will suffer from a psychosis of some sort (ONS, 2000).

Table 1: The weekly prevalence of mental health problems			
	Weekly prevalence per 1000 adults of working age	Weekly prevalence in adults of working age, per PCT of 200,000*	Weekly prevalence in adults of working age (pop 50,000,000)*
Depression	28	3,528	882,000
Mixed anxiety and depression	92	11,592	2,898,000
Anxiety disorder	47	5,922	1,480,500
Other neuroses (OCD, PD, phobias)	38	4,788	1,197,000
Psychoses	4	504	126,000
Total of all common conditions (as these often co-exist)	173	21,798	5,449,500

*assuming that 63% of the population are of working age.

OCD = obsessive compulsive disorder   PD = panic disorder

(ONS, 2000)

Ipswich, with a population of 147,000 (about 94,000 of whom are adults of working age), will have only about 375 adults of working age suffering with psychosis, but about 16,260 adults of working age with common mental health problems (ONS, 2000).

From February 2005 to September 2005, an average of 17 new referrals to the PIMHS team were being generated per week. About 36% of these came from secondary care and 64% from primary care. This means that an average of 880 referrals are made per year to the PIMHS team. This is a rate of 9.34 per thousand adults of working age per year, or 1 in 18 of those with common mental health problems.

If this data is scaled up, for an average sized PCT of 200,000 people, with around 500 people with a psychosis who receive care from specialist mental health teams (data from ONS, 2000), there will be 1,177 people of working age whose care cannot be managed with confidence in primary care but are inappropriate for specialist services.

However, this 1,177 is an estimate of the number referred to an intermediate care team only in the first year. International figures suggest that if monitoring, detection and referral of this group can be improved, then there is potentially a much larger number of patients who are not referred at present, who would benefit from referral to intermediate care. The NICE Depression Guidelines (NICE, 2004a) show that 20% of individuals with depression are still unwell two years after diagnosis. Figures from the USA suggest that with usual primary care this number is closer to 59% (Rost et al., 2002).

The impact of the PIMHS team

The impact of the PIMHS team on the number of referrals to secondary care was assessed by using routinely collected statistics from the mental health trust. The figures for new referrals to CMHTs and the crisis team were compared for the period February-May 2004 (before the service was established), and for February-May 2005 (after the service was established). The figures were available for three adjacent PCTs: Ipswich (where the PIMHS service was set up); Suffolk Coastal; and Suffolk Central. Figure 3 shows the results of the analysis:

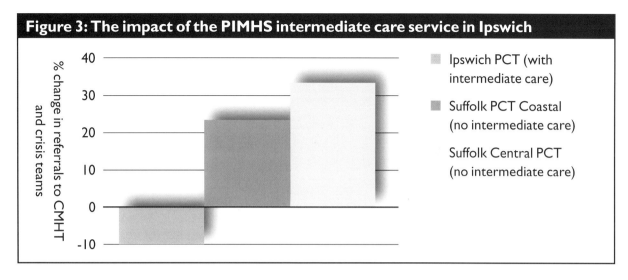

Figure 3 shows that there were 10% fewer referrals to the CMHT and crisis teams in Ipswich in the period after implementation of the service than before it was in place. However, referrals to CMHTs and crisis teams in Suffolk Coastal and Central Suffolk PCTs had increased during the period (by 23% and 33% respectively). People who were being referred to intermediate care in Ipswich in mid-2005 were still being 'inappropriately' referred to secondary care in the other two PCTs.

Independently, Ipswich Primary Care Trust, with support from its local strategic health authority, undertook an economic appraisal of the benefits of the scheme. The results suggest that there would be considerable economic and social benefit from investing in intermediate care services for those with mental health problems (Ranzetta, 2005).

CHAPTER 4

Setting up an intermediate care team

Introduction

This chapter presents a guide to setting up an intermediate care team. It is based on the experience of the Sainsbury Centre for Mental Health Intermediate Care Collaborative.

Preparation

Before work can begin to set up an intermediate care team, two key questions need to be addressed:

- What is the vision for the team? What is the overall aim?

- Who else needs to support the aim/vision that you are developing? Who are the other stakeholders? What will be their perception of what is proposed?

The people involved in this initial stage must undertake a number of preliminary tasks to ensure that the team is appropriate to the needs of the locality, and that it is supported by all those in the locality who have a stake in the provision of intermediate care. The first part of this preliminary process is identifying those stakeholders, bringing them together, and facilitating their selection of a steering group to guide the implementation of the team.

The project needs to be managed along professional lines, using tools such as needs analysis, project scoping, risk analysis, and timelines, and forming agreements on expenditure, key milestones and outcomes. Typical tools might include a project initiation document, business case document, Gantt charts and risk logs.

Identifying the stakeholders

Each locality will have a different group of stakeholders. Part of the initial process of setting up your team will be holding a preliminary meeting to identify who they are. It is very important that any relevant stakeholders are not excluded by omission.

The list below suggests those who may be present in your locality. Your stakeholder group should include a good representation from this list.

- At least two service users, who should have suffered from a common mental health problem

- Practice nurse and other members from the primary health care team

- GP

- PCT commissioner

- GP Mental Health Lead

- Local Medical Committee member

- Mental Health Trust Locality Director

- Representative from Strategic Health Authority
- CMHT manager
- CMHT worker
- Social services
- Crisis team manager/worker
- Finance advisor from the PCT
- Job Centre Plus representative
- Representatives from voluntary organisations – especially those offering benefit, debt and employment advice
- Representatives from local minority ethnic organisations and community projects
- Representatives from primary care counselling
- Representatives from primary care psychology
- Mental health trust psychologist
- Consultant psychiatrist.

Not every part of the country will have all of these groups. The intention is that those stakeholders who are present in your area are invited; it may be that in some areas, there are other stakeholders specific to your locality, who should also be included.

Once the stakeholders have all been identified, then a simple 'stakeholder register' can be maintained by the project manager (see 'Appointing a project manager' later in this chapter). This helps to ensure that stakeholders are not 'excluded by omission' from participation in the project.

Focus groups of these stakeholders can be formed, or interviews conducted, to explore issues such as:

- The quality of existing services
- The range of local provision (statutory and non-statutory)
- Gaps in provision
- Service user and carer experiences
- The nature of service relationships and partnerships.

Forming a steering group

Once the stakeholders have been identified, they should hold a meeting to agree on a core steering group that they are happy is representative of the locality.

The steering group needs to meet on a regular basis to oversee the development of the service. It is vital that the core group has the authority to see the project through, and it will need to report on a regular basis to the Primary Care Trust Professional Executive Committee (PCT PEC) and Board. They must establish clear lines of accountability and reporting at an early stage, and ensure that the project has the active support of the Local Implementation Team (LIT), PCT Chief Executive and Finance Director.

Appointing a project manager

The core group would benefit from a professional project manager to oversee the development of the scheme, along established project management lines. The project manager is responsible for making appropriate reports to the stakeholders, and also for ensuring that action points are carried out. When the project becomes operational it is likely that the service manager will naturally take on the project management role.

Supporting the project manager appropriately is vital. They will need regular contact with the responsible director (or a senior manager with clearly defined authority), Mental Health Lead, and also with a representative from the finance department (unless this role is taken by the director).

The trio of PCT director/manager, Mental Health Lead, and service manager/project manager provides an ideal group to oversee day to day development. The smooth functioning of this group is one of the key attributes for success.

Developing an evaluation tool

■ How do you know that the team is working properly? How can you evaluate the team, clinically and managerially?

An evaluation tool should be developed in the early stages of setting up an intermediate care team. Chapter 6 provides guidelines for evaluating the team's effectiveness.

Implementation

The process of setting up an intermediate care team involves a number of initial processes: identifying the client group for the service; identifying the team members; setting up the team and bringing the team members together in partnership.

Identifying the client group in your locality

■ What tasks need to be done by GPs, PCTs and others to find out how many people there are in the locality with complex and enduring common mental health problems that fit the criteria for intermediate care?

The exercises in Chapter 5 should be completed by the relevant stakeholders. The steering committee should then meet to examine the figures and ascertain the client group for intermediate care within the locality.

Identifying the team members

■ Who should be in the team to cater for the needs identified within the locality?

■ Who is available locally who could be in the team? Who employs them? How can the stakeholders work together towards managing this group of people?

The precise composition of the team depends on the needs that you have identified for your locality, and the resources that you have available. The following may be included in the team:

• **Experts by experience** (including 'expert patients') could be used for telephone follow up, seeing patients in clinics, or to act as friends or buddies to accompany clients to appointments.

• **Practitioners (GPs or nurses) with a special interest (PwSI)** provide a strong medical presence, vital to give medication advice. Often clients will have had several courses of medication, and these practitioners need to be of sufficient experience to be able to provide advice about more specialised medication to the rest of the team, and to referrers.

- **Primary care mental health workers** – the basic workers in the team, providing assessments of new clients, and acting as case managers and therapists, within their experience. They also provide a link working role between primary and secondary care, and act as mentors to graduate primary care mental health workers. These workers may come from diverse backgrounds. They should have experience in delivering the briefer mental health interventions that are going to be of value to this client group. It is not necessary for them to have direct primary care experience, but if they do not then 'adaptability' should be one of their characteristics. Time will need to be put aside for them to be educated about the differences and to allow them to change their practice over time. This time will be shorter if they have some experience in link working, or direct work in primary care. These workers could be nurses, occupational therapists or social workers.

- **Graduate primary care mental health workers** – often less experienced clinically, but able to oversee less intensive therapies, such as guided bibliotherapy, or computerised cognitive behavioural therapy (CBT). As they gain experience, they will also be able to facilitate groups. They can act as 'buddies' to accompany clients to appointments.

- **Gateway workers** – probably performing the same functions as the primary mental health workers, but these workers have a specific function in the NSF-MH (DH, 1999), and the initial intention in the NSF was that funding would be provided for 500 Gateway Workers in total across the country, by 2004.

- **Black and minority ethnic (BME) workers**, as appropriate to the area.

- **People working in partner organisations**:
  - Job Centre Plus – to fast track clients with mental health problems
  - Citizens Advice Bureau workers – debt, benefit and legal advice
  - Housing – often the busiest workers
  - Benefit advice
  - Advocacy
  - Volunteers to act as 'buddies' – a vital function as simple 'signposting' may fail due to anxiety; arranging to accompany the client to an appointment may greatly enhance the effectiveness of signposting.

- **Administrative support staff** – this work is key to the success of the team; it is a false economy using clinical staff to perform these functions.

- **Counsellors** – may be provided from the counselling service already available.

- **Therapists and psychologists** – CBT is a key therapy in the NICE anxiety and depression guidelines (NICE, 2004a, 2004b). Delivery of CBT in intermediate care means that patients are able to access it rapidly.

The steering group will now need to look at who is already working in the locality who could come to work for the team. All the available workers in the groups should be included – enquiries need to be made of all the organisations identified as stakeholders, with reference to the stakeholder register. The assessment should be undertaken by members of the steering group, and the results should be discussed at a steering group meeting.

Table 2 shows an example of a worker log to be filled in by the members of the steering group. It shows four locations. The table should be amended to show the number of locations relevant to your locality. The number of each type of worker in each location should be entered and totalled.

Table 2: Assessing people currently working in the locality who could become part of the intermediate care team

Type of worker	Location 1	Location 2	Location 3	Location 4	Total
Expert by experience					
PwSI					
Primary Care MH Worker – nurse					
Primary Care MH Worker – OT					
Primary Care MH Worker – SW					
Graduate primary care mental health workers					
Gateway worker					
Job Centre Plus					
BME workers					
Citizens Advice					
Housing					
Benefit advice					
Advocacy					
Volunteers					
Administrative staff					
Counsellors					
Psychological therapists					

Bringing the team together – making partnership work

■ How can the team be brought together? What will work locally?

No single professional (from whatever background) could provide all the care needed for those in the client group for intermediate care, as their needs cover several different care groups including health, social care, housing and employment. An intermediate care team is likely to be made up of workers with experience of working in many different cultures of care. Workers will have to develop entirely new ways of working appropriate to the intermediate care team, to cope with the likely workload, which may be considerably more than some of the staff members may have experienced before, and allow clients to be seen by those who can best help them, with the time available to do so. The workers will have to borrow ways of working from primary and secondary care, and the voluntary sector. This means a change in philosophy from 'having a case load', to 'doing today's work today', and delegating responsibility for appointments and waiting times to other staff. This is accompanied by giving clear 'safety net' instructions to patients, to ensure that they know what action to take if their condition deteriorates.

Workers will also need to learn to work in partnership with each other. Specialist mental health services such as community mental health teams (CMHTs) have been aware of the need for a holistic approach for the people for whom they care, and have extensive experience of working in a partnership. The same is true for the other care groups. Partnership is a much explored concept within the health and social care sectors, and as such there is plenty of experience to show what makes an effective partnership.

A previous publication from the Sainsbury Centre for Mental Health, *Taking your Partners: Using opportunities for inter-agency partnership in mental health* (SCMH, 2000), explored partnership working in some detail. Within that publication was a checklist to ensure effective partnership. The following is an amended version of that checklist to use to facilitate and assess partnership working within your intermediate care team. These questions can be reviewed at various times throughout the project to assess the development of the team, and the strengths of bringing different partners together.

▶ Are the strategic objectives of the team clear and agreed?

There is little point in embarking on a significant work programme unless the objectives, in terms of the outcomes for services and service users, are clear. Joint working is a means to an end and not an outcome in itself.

Intermediate care has specific and achievable objectives, agreed by stakeholders. It is focused on developing a new team, drawn from existing resources, if these are adequate, that provides care for people with mental health problems who cannot be managed with confidence in primary care, but are inappropriate for secondary care.

▶ Do the different services involved in the team share boundaries and working areas – are they 'coterminous'?

Answering this question requires a review of what community resources are available, from health care, social care, housing, employment, the voluntary sector, and the user and carer movements. Do they all share the same boundaries? Boundaries may not only be geographical, but can relate to age, type of disorder, ethnicity or other modality [criterion]. During the detailed implementation phase of the project, these areas of coterminosity need to be explored and agreed amongst all partners. If any gaps in coterminosity are identified, joint working arrangements need to be identified to fill in the gaps.

▶ Is the leadership of the team creative and entrepreneurial? Is everyone involved signed up to change?

Who is driving the agenda – why is there a need for the service? Is the development being led by clinicians, or managers, or users and carers? Is the incentive for change about clinical service development, or is it financial (e.g. practice based commissioning)? Is there an individual within the organisation who is going to make the changes happen? Is that individual at the right place within the commissioning organisation, where he/she has authority to make decisions? Is he/she likely to remain in post in the short term and if not who will continue to own the process?

▶ Is there a reasonable history of successful joint working among the sectors making up your team's workforce?

Is there a specific history of good or bad relations between various sectors that is going to influence the outcome? For example, how well do primary and secondary care mental health services get on – is there a shared understanding of their respective roles? Is there a fear that the new team will leach expert resources from secondary care to primary care for example, or a fear that secondary care will use the new team as a step down from CMHTs?

▶ How will you ensure good communication between the stakeholders in the team?

What processes will be put in place to ensure that the various stakeholders are aware of what is being proposed, and what the benefits are likely to be? More specifically, how will the new team share clinical data with the various sectors who are contributing resources? How will outcomes be assessed? How will a commissioner know if this service is 'cost effective'?

▶ **What agreed outcome measures or indicators will you use to monitor the success of the team?**

See Chapter 6 for a detailed review of the evaluation process, and shared outcomes.

▶ **Is the team focused on its 'consumers' i.e. the client group for intermediate care? Are they sufficiently involved in the project?**

Involving the user and carer movement in the development of this project is essential. However it is equally important to ensure that the correct groups of users and carers are appropriately involved – the type of people who are most likely to benefit from this intervention, are, by definition, not those who have used specialist mental health services extensively. Therefore there is a need to ensure that users and carers are actively engaged who have experience of primary care services, but not extensive experience of specialist mental health services.

▶ **Is there planning in place for a shared training strategy?**

As the project develops, the training agenda for a number of professionals, within the team, and within primary and secondary care, will become clear. This needs to be developed into a shared training strategy.

▶ **Do the team members understand and respect each others' working cultures?**

It is essential that local authority colleagues understand the NHS culture, which is strongly centrally driven, and that NHS colleagues understand the local agenda of local authorities. This requires mutual respect and accommodation e.g. NHS colleagues being willing to work to convince local politicians of the need for change, and local authority colleagues understanding the role of central guidance and regional performance management in the NHS.

This is a continuing issue, but as the various modernisation agendas develop across PCTs and local authorities, they converge, and organisations are much more aware of each other's culture. However, by being aware of possible problems at an early stage in the implementation of your intermediate care team, some of the potential for misunderstanding can be avoided.

▶ **Are the relevant senior clinicians and practitioners engaged in the process?**

Engaging general practitioners is central to this programme, but since it is designed to increase the service available to patients who otherwise would not receive such care, involving GPs is not necessarily a major issue. Likewise engaging a psychiatrist to provide support would be valuable. Engaging some individuals may be difficult and a separate strategy may be required for dealing with this situation. Other senior professionals who contribute significantly but are much easier to engage are social workers and nurses, as well as the various new community workers such as graduate mental health workers. All these clinicians need not only to be engaged, but to act as leaders for the programme.

The intermediate care team in practice

The initial phase of the team's existence needs to allow for a 'bedding-in' period of a few weeks to allow policies to be written, accommodation arranged, and basics such as office furnishing, computers, faxes and telephones etc. to be properly managed. Failure to do this will have an enduring effect on the functioning of the team. The team will need facilities to enable it to consult at a rate consistent with the expected workload.

It may be sensible to phase the appointments of the workers, so that the team manager and administrative staff start several weeks before the rest of the workers.

This early phase of the team also involves developing and testing the systems to be put in practice, including the referral process, the appointments system, records storage and archiving, and the assessment process. The rest of this chapter explores two main components of this development and testing process – referral and assessment.

The referral process

The team needs to be advertised to the referrers, and stationery such as referral forms should be designed and distributed. The mechanisms of referral should be subject to a 'dry run' to ensure safety. For example, do you wish faxes to be received in an empty building? If not, does the fax machine have sufficient memory to manage if you remove the paper every night?

Questions to consider when developing the referral process include:

- Will you use a referral form?
- Will referrers post, fax or email it?
- What details will it contain?
- How will you produce the form?
- How will you distribute it?

From the beginning you will need to design a system to receive and manage the referrals:

- Do you send appointments out on receipt of the referral?
- Do you expect clients to phone in to arrange the appointment?
- Do clients have to return a letter or card before you send them an appointment? (opting in)
- What will the team policy be on failure to attend?
- What will the team policy be on failure to respond to communication?
- Do referrers give clients an explanatory leaflet on referral?
- How long will an assessment appointment be?
- How long will a review appointment be?
- How many sessions will you expect the clients to be seen for?

You will also need to decide locally on who can refer to the team. This may include:

- GPs
- Patients themselves
- Practice nurses
- Crisis team
- Counsellors
- A&E
- Job Centre Plus
- CMHT
- Acute hospital wards.

The referral form used in a working intermediate care team, PIMHS in Ipswich, is included as an example of the referral process (Figure 4).

Figure 4: An example of a referral form from the PIMHS intermediate care team in Ipswich

PIMHS referral form
Primary Care Intermediate Mental Health Service

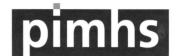

Please FAX this form to PIMHS

Miss ❏ Ms ❏ Mrs ❏ Mr ❏ Name: Date of Birth:	Client ID Number: *(PIMHS use only)*
	Client's preferred telephone contact:
Address: Postcode:	All current prescribed drugs:
Presenting problem: *DASS scores (if done):*	Results of investigations (eg thyroid, liver/gamma GT, MCV etc if done):
	Usual GP and Practice:

Relevant past medical history (previous mental disorder, current physical illnesses/disabilities and drug treatments so far. *Computer generated summaries are acceptable*):

Other interventions: *(please tick)*

1. ❏ Self-help literature (what?)   2. ❏ Counselling (who?)   3. ❏ Anxiety management (where?)

....

Additional needs/issues: *(please tick)*	1. ❏ Financial 2. ❏ Employment	3. ❏ Housing 4. ❏ Relationships	5. ❏ Illness 6. ❏ Other ....

	Interpreter required?: ❏ Yes ❏ No
  Signed: Date:	If Yes, please specify which language ....

PRF Version 1/Jan 05

The assessment process

The assessment is the initial interview at which the client's problem is discussed with a mental health worker, and the worker and client agree a working diagnosis, and a shared management plan, completion of which will hopefully lead to resolution of the difficulties.

Questions to consider when developing the assessment process include:

- Will you use a standardised assessment tool?

- Will this be the same as that used by your CMHT?

- What rating scales will you use?

- If you use scales, will others understand them?

- What risk assessment will you use?

- Will the other teams in your locality accept an assessment from your team, or will the client have to be re-assessed on onward referral?

- How long will an assessment take?

- How many workers should do an assessment?

- How experienced should those assessing be? (It may be appropriate to ensure that a robust, holistic assessment is done initially by a very experienced worker.)

- Will you aim to assess quickly, then assign patients to wait for treatment, or assess and treat in strict order of referral, more slowly?

CHAPTER 5

Assessing the need for intermediate care in your locality

Introduction

Establishing the need for intermediate care and the local service gap it will fill is essential. Intermediate care teams are designed, among other things, to fill the gap between primary and secondary care and to intervene early and holistically to reduce pressure on secondary care. A needs assessment therefore describes the gap and likely volume of activity in order to establish the required resource. A more complete description should indicate the nature of skill mix for the intermediate care team, and the partnerships it needs to form that will be key to its success. The needs assessment also crucially provides a baseline against which the extent of change can be measured.

A needs assessment will help in:

- establishing the strengths and weaknesses of local provision

- describing what services are available in the community (sometimes called a service map)

- describing gaps in service and the resource that would be used to fill these

- describing the target group(s) for an intermediate care team

- exposing weaknesses in local statistical data and other potential evidence sources

- giving consideration to the funding of the team, including any savings an intermediate care team could produce

- defining the objectives for the team and how these should be measured

- providing a baseline from which to measure progress, impact and change

- forming the questions and hypothesis for the later evaluation.

This chapter is divided into two main areas. The first shows how to estimate the prevalence of all mental health problems in your locality, from the perspective of either a whole PCT, or an individual GP practice. The second gives suggestions for how to estimate the number of people with a common mental health condition whose problem is complex and enduring, and who are therefore part of the client group for intermediate care.

One of the first stages of setting up an intermediate care team is to set up a steering group of the stakeholders involved in your team (see Chapter 4). These exercises should be completed by as many of the appropriate stakeholders in the team as possible, and then presented at a steering group meeting. From this, the stakeholders will gain valuable insight into the needs and problems of the locality, viewed from different perspectives.

The prevalence of mental illness in a locality

This section is designed to provide you with an estimate of the number of people in your locality who have mental health problems. It is split up into two exercises, one for PCTs to complete, and one for an individual GP practice.

Incidence of mental illness within a PCT

Tables 3 and 4 can be used to manually calculate the approximate incidence of mental health problems in your PCT, among people aged 16 to 64, per week.

You will first need to fill out Table 3 with the following information (from the Department of Health website at www.dh.gov.uk): the total population in your PCT; the percentage of people within the PCT who are aged from 16-64; the number of people in the PCT in this age range (worked out from the percentage); this number divided by 1,000; and the Mental Health Index in your PCT area. We have used the Mental Illness Needs Index 2000 (MINI2K). This will either be above or below 1.0. A figure below 1.0 indicates that the area is less needy (from a mental health perspective) than the national average, and a figure above 1.0 indicates greater mental health needs.

Table 3				
Population in your PCT	Percentage of people aged 16-64 in PCT	Number of people aged 16-64 in PCT	Number of people aged 16-64 divided by 1000	Mental Illness Needs Index (MINI2K) in your PCT

The data from Table 3 should be used to fill out Table 4. Column 1 in Table 4 gives the weekly prevalence of each type of mental illness per 1,000 people, using the Office for National Statistics report *Psychiatric Morbidity among adults living in private households* data (ONS, 2000). The common mental health conditions of depression and anxiety often co-exist – the figure for 'all neuroses' allows for this. To complete column 2, multiply the number of people aged 16-64 per 1000 people in your PCT (column 4 in Table 3) by the prevalence per 1,000 of each type of mental illness.

Filling out column 2 gives an average rate of each type of mental illness based on the prevalence of that mental illness averaged across the UK. Completing column 3 will give you a clearer idea of the situation in your own locality, by weighting the national average by the local circumstances in your PCT. To fill out this column, multiply the figure in column 2 by the Mental Illness Needs Index of your PCT (column 5 in Table 3).

Table 4			
Diagnosis	**Weekly prevalence per 1,000 adults aged 16-64**	**Prevalence multiplied by population**	**Population prevalence adjusted by Mental Illness Needs Index (MINI2K)**
Psychotic illness	4		
Mixed anxiety and depression	92		
Generalised anxiety	47		
Depressive episode	28		
All phobias	19		
Obsessive compulsive disorder	12		
Panic disorder	7		
All neuroses	173		
Drug dependence	42		
Alcohol dependence	81		

Tables 3 and 4 can also be converted into a template for a spreadsheet. A sample spreadsheet using 2002 data is available on the SCMH website at www.scmh.org.uk/icc. Up-to-date data for filling out the spreadsheet – on PCT population, percentage of people in your PCT aged 16-64, and Mental Illness Needs Index – can be found on the Department of Health website (www.dh.gov.uk).

Incidence of mental illness within a GP practice

Several different approaches can be used to complete this task.

1. Computer search

The most obvious is to conduct a computer search for the diagnoses of all patients registered with the practice – but unless the practice has been disciplined in using agreed Read codes (for recording diagnoses and treatment in primary care) it is likely that the data entry will be inaccurate – it is also difficult to know whether someone is still ill or has recovered. Another approach is to search medication records for medications used for anxiety and depression but these have many different uses, so this method is likely to lead to inaccuracies too. For all these reasons, unless you are very sure about the data quality, this is not a method we can recommend.

However, if you are able to do this accurately you could also look further at how many people suffering with these conditions have had two or more treatments for them, and still appear to be suffering, in the last year. Also look for those with co-existing physical diseases, who have had one intervention for their mental health condition, which has failed.

2. Population estimate

The next is to simply use the data on the prevalence of different types of common mental illness from the ONS 2000 *Survey of psychiatric morbidity* to provide a rough estimate for your practice. If you wish you can further refine the estimate by multiplying it by the Mental Illness Needs Index. This method will be rapid, but will be inaccurate if your practice has anything other than an 'average' population.

Tables 5 and 6 can be used to manually calculate the approximate prevelance of common mental health problems in your practice, among working age adults (aged 16-64), per week. They can be used as a template for a spreadsheet. You will need to enter your practice's population, the percentage of people aged 16-64, and the Mental Illness Needs Index (MINI2K) for your practice (available on the Department of Health website at www.dh.gov.uk) into the spreadsheet.

Table 5

Population in your practice	Percentage of people aged 16-64 in practice	Number of people aged 16-64 in practice	Number of people aged 16-64 divided by 1000	Mental Illness Needs Index (MINI2K) in practice

Table 6

Diagnosis	Weekly prevalence per 1,000 adults aged 16-64	Prevalence multiplied by practice population	Population prevalence adjusted by Mental Illness Needs Index (MINI2K)
Psychotic illness	4		
Mixed anxiety and depression	92		
Generalised anxiety	47		
Depressive episode	28		
All phobias	19		
Obsessive compulsive disorder	12		
Panic disorder	7		
All neuroses	173		
Drug dependence	42		
Alcohol dependence	81		

3. 'Slogger Sheet'

The clinician simply records on a sheet their perception of the broad diagnostic category that best fits the patient. Table 7 is an example of a sheet of this type.

The table should be completed by every clinician for one week, and then totalled, providing the expected number of individuals with each type of diagnosis, per week, for your practice. The method is simple, but can clearly mis-estimate rare conditions. It is also dependent on the clinician's ability to recognise the conditions, with ability on the first consultation varying from 20 to 80%, and averaging 50% (Goldberg & Huxley, 1992; Kessler et al., 1999).

Table 7						
Patient No.	Age	Sex	Diagnostic Category*	How many treatments in last year?	Still actively suffering?	Co-existing physical disease?

* Enter into this column one of the following five numbers to denote diagnostic category:

1 anxiety

2 anxiety/depression

3 depression

4 schizophrenia

5 bipolar

To complete this process, you will need to perform a basic calculation to give the weekly prevalence per 1000 adults of working age:

1. Add up the number of adults of working age seen with **each condition individually** in one week.

2. Add up the **total** number of adults of working age seen in the week.

3. Divide the number suffering with a condition by the total number seen. This is the weekly prevalence.

4. Multiply this number by 1,000 to obtain the weekly prevalence per 1,000 adults of working age.

This figure can then be used to estimate the weekly prevalence of conditions in a population by simply scaling the number up. However, the figures reached by using this method are very dependent on the clinician's ability to detect mental illness, and the particular client group seen that week, so they are somewhat subjective.

The need for intermediate care

Many people with common mental health problems are wholly, and successfully, treated in primary care. The calculations previously undertaken in this chapter include this group – people whose common mental health problems are not complex, and whose needs are catered for within primary care. To estimate the demand for intermediate care in your PCT or GP practice, you will therefore need to estimate the number of people whose needs are complex and enduring, and cannot be dealt with successfully in primary care alone. This section provides a number of suggestions for estimating this need.

The reason for doing this work is that it is likely that most of the patients not accepted for specialist care will be suitable for intermediate care.

The usefulness of the following exercises is multiplied if they are performed and then the results of as many as possible presented to a stakeholder meeting. This will be one of the key meetings in the development of an intermediate care service, as the stakeholders will develop a shared understanding of the true amount of unmet need and suffering.

Incidence of common mental health problems with complex needs

There are a number of ways of calculating the incidence of common mental health problems with complex needs in a locality.

'Slogger sheet'

This is best completed in each individual GP practice with a 'slogger sheet'. If a PCT wanted to make an estimate of patients with complex needs across the locality, they could ask a number of practices to complete the sheets, and extrapolate the data for the whole PCT from this. Each practitioner in a practice can use the table to record numbers of patients with either anxiety or depression, who also have needs that cannot be met by primary care alone. Table 8 provides an example of a 'slogger sheet' for this process. The clinician should simply tick whichever of the problems applies to each patient.

Table 8			Type of problem							
Patient identifier	No of treatments in primary care	Housing problem	Work or unemployment problem	Benefit problem	Drug or alcohol problem	Previous abuse	BME/ Refugee	Domestic violence	Other issues

Other indicators of incidence of common mental health problems with complex needs

The following exercises will help to build up a picture of the need for intermediate care in a locality, from the point of view of secondary care services. They focus on ascertaining the number of people who are seen by secondary care services and then advised that the system cannot help them, despite their distress.

■ **The number of 'inappropriate' referrals to your CMHT**
How many people are referred to your CMHT, and either not seen, or referred back immediately following assessment? Your CMHT manager should be able to provide these figures for you. If they are unable to provide this information, then speak to the Director of Commissioning, as this is basic data on the quality and quantity of care that is being provided which is essential to an effective organisation. People in this 'inappropriate referral category' are often suffering with common mental health problems with complex needs.

■ **The number of 'inappropriate' referrals to your crisis team**
How many people are referred to your crisis team, and either not seen, or referred back immediately following assessment? Your crisis team manager should be able to provide these figures for you.

■ **Attendance statistics at A&E and number of mental health assessments**
Many people attend Accident and Emergency with deliberate self harm, or other symptoms of distress. Some of these people will be assessed by mental health professionals at the request of the A&E staff. The numbers of people attending with psychological symptoms, the numbers assessed, and the

numbers of those assessed on whom no action is taken can all help throw light on the scale of the problem.

■ **The number of admissions to psychiatric facilities**
This can be collected as a baseline measurement that again illustrates the extent of the problem. If possible try to separate out those with common mental health problems from those with severe and enduring mental health problems.

Population estimate of somatisation within a PCT

Patients presenting with physical symptoms, but no detectable physical condition, form a large part of the client base for intermediate care. Table 9 will help you to find out how many people are likely to suffer with medically unexplained symptoms in your PCT, and how much their care costs.

To complete this table, you will need to know the number of new episodes of each type of outpatient 'new referral' listed which are contracted for in your PCT every year. You can find this out by contacting your PCT commissioners or finance department. This data should be entered into column 1. Column 2 provides an estimate of the fraction of patients attending each type of outpatient clinics, with no detectable physical illness (Bass, 2003, Nimnuan et al., 2000), and column 3 will give you an estimated figure of such patients in your own PCT. To fill out column 3, multiply the figures in column 1 by the figures in column 2. Column 4 will provide you with the estimated cost of patients with somatisation to your PCT annually. To fill this out, multiply the figures in column 3 by £955 – an estimate of the cost of resource use by each patient with somatisation (Reid et al., 2001).

Table 9				
	Column 1	**Column 2**	**Column 3**	**Column 4**
Speciality	**Number of new episodes contracted for in your PCT annually**	**Estimated proportion with no detectable physical illness**	**Estimated number of patients with somatisation in each field**	**Cost to PCT based on per head cost of £955 (as per Reid et al., 2002)**
Cardiology		0.5		
Gastroenterology		0.5		
Neurology		0.5		
Dental		0.5		
Gynaecology		0.5		
Other medical		0.3		
Totals				

Somatisation: A GP's personal perpective

This section, written by a family doctor, gives a personal perspective on how to estimate the incidence of somatisation in an individual GP practice.

Background

As a general practitioner, I have always had a particular interest in mental health problems manifesting themselves as medically unexplained symptoms. Over my seven years as a Principal in General Practice, I have become somewhat frustrated by my inability to help patients with strange symptom sets that have defied treatment, investigation and ultimately any definitive resolution.

In the course of a typical consulting day I expect to see at least two to three patients presenting with medically unexplained symptoms. This makes me feel confused, disempowered and rather helpless. I have tended, in the past, to 'tactically' resolve these consultations by collusion which, in practical terms, means offering another referral, review of treatment or investigation. 'Biting the bullet' and being candid about how I feel with the patient has borne fruit but usually ends up with recrimination, denial and rejection by the latter.

Recent changes in my own career have, however, led me to realise that this is a problem which must be tackled. Through my work as Clinical Mental Health Lead for my primary care trust, I have realised, through numerous discussions with peers and colleagues, that my experience of the needs and challenges of this group of patients is very common. In my role as case-reviewer, I have also undertaken tasks usually delegated to others – notes summarisation for either the nGMS GP Contract or in preparation for Deanery training accreditation. Looking through these notes I picked up several key characteristics which helped me to 'profile' those with medically unexplained symptoms. I also realised that these patients had often experienced a fairly prodigious 'career' through secondary care, with no resolution or improvement in symptoms – there is an appreciable financial imperative for primary care trusts to manage somatisation disorder effectively.

To estimate the true volume of the client group in my own practice, I devised a calculation based on this experience, which can be used in other practices.

Identifying the 'prescribing profile'

The basis of the technique is similar to one that was used locally (and probably commonly elsewhere) to generate the Seriously Mentally Ill Registers for nGMS – it is based on identifying repeat prescribing. I looked at which categories of drugs tended to appear, and identified the following features in those with medically unexplained symptoms:

1) Antidepressant medication had been prescribed by a variety of practitioners spanning primary and secondary care, to almost every one of these patients. Some of this was a genuine attempt to broach and pay homage to the subject of underlying mental health problems. Most however, and I am as guilty of this as anybody, were presented to the patient as a panacea for their symptoms with no mention of their mental health as a factor.

2) Most patients had also been prescribed at least one symptomatic treatment. These included 'pain killers' – largely non steroidal anti-inflammatory drugs (NSAIDs, or aspirin-like drugs used for pain and inflammation), opiates (codeine- or morphine-like drugs) or combination preparations, usually a combination of paracetamol with an opiate (e.g. co-proxamol), in isolation or mixed with each other. Hypnotics (sleeping tablets), especially benzodiazepines, were very common. Finally, many drugs for abdominal discomfort (largely antispasmodics such as mebeverine and hyoscine butyl bromide but also drugs for sickness or nausea, such as prochlorperazine) were also present.

Gathering the data and the calculation

The aim of producing this 'prescribing profile' is to use it to produce a workable list of patients – a quasi disease register. The practice computer software can be used to identify the number of patients who fulfil these criteria. The following is a step-by-step guide to creating this list. Slightly more advanced, but still fairly easy, is generating a list of names. In essence:

1. Identify those patients with repeat prescriptions for antidepressant medication.

2. From this group, identify those with active or recent repeats of any of the following:
   a. Hypnotics (sleeping tablets)
   b. Symptomatic Gastro-Intestinal treatments (drugs for abdominal discomfort)
   c. Analgesics (Pain killers) (NSAIDs or Opiates or Combinations).

3. Identify which of these patients are receiving palliative care for a terminal illness and delete them from the list.

4. Multiply the final number (i.e. the number of patients on antidepressants, minus the number not on symptomatic medications, minus the number on palliative care) by £955 (Reid *et al.*, 2002) to estimate the cost of these patients' care to a practice.

The results

Using this calculation, I identified 113 of 3,668 (3%) patients in my practice list. You could also use this method to create a list of names of patients who fulfil all these criteria.

My practice patient demographics are not too different from the Waltham Forest PCT population. I therefore extrapolated the figures across the PCT giving a total of 7,701 patients with medically unexplained symptoms. The estimated mean cost to the health care economy per patient per year of patients with medically unexplained symptoms is £955, most of which is unnecessary admission and investigation (Reid *et al.*, 2002) – the costs are staggering, running into millions of pounds per PCT.

The extrapolation makes big assumptions but highlights the order of magnitude that we are dealing with. This is a cost we cannot ignore.

By Dr Shahid Dadabhoy
Family Practitioner, Chingford, London
Professional Executive Committee Mental Health Lead, Waltham Forest PCT

CHAPTER 6

Evaluating intermediate care

Introduction

Evaluation is not a specific methodology or set of methods – evaluations can utilise a variety of research methods – but rather as Robson (2002) states, it is the purpose or objective of an exercise that defines it as an evaluation. Evaluations are particularly important for assessing the worth of new or innovative projects, and an evaluation is an essential part of establishing an intermediate care team.

All too often evaluations are an afterthought, commissioned after the launch of a service at a time when commissioners need to decide on future funding. Evaluation needs to form part of the earliest thinking about launching a new service. Where possible, the information to be collected for the evaluation should form part of the service's routine data collection, for example for the purposes of measuring outcomes. This creates a capacity in a team to conduct audits and ongoing monitoring and reduces both the cost and effort of any evaluation.

Evaluating intermediate care

The *National Service Framework for Mental Health* (DH, 1999) is quite prescriptive in parts, describing the role, function and even make-up of new services. Intermediate care is not such a prescribed service and in a restricted financial climate such services need to demonstrate their impact and in particular that they:

- represent value for money

- have an impact on a wider system and ideally can produce savings

- are clinically effective

- produce other benefits to service users (e.g. a return to economic activity or other proxies of an improved quality of life)

- represent a service improvement.

Evaluation of your intermediate care service will provide you with the information to prove that the service fulfils all these requirements.

The evaluation should ideally be in two stages: a needs assessment before the launch of the service, and a main evaluation after the service has launched.

The needs assessment

Stage one is a needs assessment that commences before any service is launched. It establishes the case for that service and the nature of its resource. The needs assessment process is described in Chapter 5. An additional reason for conducting the needs assessment is to prepare the ground for the main evaluation. For example, if existing information systems and routine data collection will not adequately answer the main evaluation questions, the needs assessment provides an early warning of this, and recommendations on how to rectify it.

The main evaluation

Stage two is the main evaluation, taking place after the service has launched, with most of its activity taking place once the team has been established.

The main evaluation is defined by the needs assessment. This will identify the questions the main evaluation should address in gauging the success of the intermediate care team. Box 3 provides an example of an evaluation hypothesis and the questions for an intermediate care evaluation.

Box 3: The proposed evaluation of the Ipswich intermediate care team

Hypothesis: that intermediate care will improve the mental health of people with identified low-level depression and complex needs, thereby reducing the global demands such people make of health and other services.

Evaluation questions:

1. Does intermediate care have an impact on people referred with depression, stress and anxiety?

2. Are clients satisfied with the service?

3. Are GPs satisfied with the service?

4. Are the number of 'inappropriate' referrals reduced?

5. What are the number of complex mental health related presentations to GPs (also useful question for needs assessment)?

6. What is the impact of intermediate care on mental health services?

7. What is the impact on other agencies?

8. What are the factors influencing intermediate care success (client and professional perspectives)?

The evaluation should run alongside the new service ensuring that data is collected and inputted throughout the course of the evaluation. Some of the information collection processes suggested in the rest of this chapter should take place at regular intervals and others should be implemented once the intermediate care team is well established.

The main evaluation may choose as part of its process to follow a particular set of 'service users' (perhaps a random sample) to provide the most detailed picture, but some basic statistics should be collected on all service users.

The main evaluation will repeat some of the elements of the needs assessment, such as interviews and focus groups, but this time exploring any impact the introduction of intermediate care has had. It is unlikely that a realistic idea of the impact can be gauged much before a year after launch, as most new services need time to 'bed-in' and establish themselves.

A number of data collection methods are appropriate for evaluating intermediate care. As different intermediate care teams may vary in their design to suit a given locality, so too should the methods of collecting evidence for the evaluation. Whatever evaluation design is ultimately settled on, it is advisable to consider a range of methods, both qualitative and quantitative. This will help to reduce the risk posed by over-dependence on a particular method (that could prove difficult to employ), but more importantly no single method is likely to address all the questions in an intermediate care team evaluation. Additionally, findings from one source or method can be tested against findings from others, and as such are likely to create greater confidence in the evaluation's outcome.

For all the different data collection processes, considerable forethought and preparation are required. For example in order to demonstrate any wider impact of intermediate care, consideration should be given to collecting data from other agencies. This would require developing an agreement with any such agency and tackling all the ethical issues that this would raise including seeking the informed consent of the service user.

Suggested main evaluation information collection processes include:

- **Hard data collected at intervals** to gauge impact of interventions, for example service referral/use statistics; rating scales to demonstrate clinical improvement; and details of critical events, for example admissions to hospital and use of primary care. Incorporating as much of this data collection into routine practice would reduce the 'burden' of the evaluation on the team once launched. Additionally a database that incorporates the different data needs to be developed.

- **Qualitative data collected at intervals** to gauge impact of the intervention. Service users and carers may be interviewed throughout the course of the intervention possibly pre- but certainly post-intervention. Professional and other perspectives may be better collected when the service is well established, preferably at least a year after launch (through interviews and focus groups).

- **Satisfaction of service users** tested through a specially designed questionnaire and through interviews. This would be conducted after a course of treatment has been completed.

- **Satisfaction of key professionals (e.g. GPs)** tested through a specially designed questionnaire and also through interviews. This could concern GP satisfaction with the service provided to particular service users and be conducted after an intervention, or seek more general impressions once the service has been established.

- **Data from other agencies** should be collected, where possible, to explore the wider impact of intermediate care for example on housing, uptake of Incapacity Benefit and work. Essentially data would be collected on individual clients on their pre- and post-intervention state/circumstances (but will most likely be collected retrospectively in both cases). This would require agreements and consideration of ethical issues. It would be collected throughout the evaluation.

- **Workshops** should be held at critical points to present findings and work collaboratively on solutions. The workshops could be drawn from the broad group of stakeholders who took part in the interviews or focus group.

Analysis

The analysis will be dictated by the questions that you wish to have answered, and the methods that you have used to collect data. Of especial importance is whether you are able to compare baseline data (before the service was set up – possibly from the needs assessment), with data once the service is up and running. Once you have the data you will be able to conduct a statistical analysis, to show significant differences, or associations. You could conduct qualitative analysis using interviews or focus groups, workshops, or free text questionnaires. This will help you search for themes and common issues.

It is not appropriate in the limited space here to describe the likely analytical processes for each of the above and it is recommended that those with some expertise in such analysis be engaged for the task.

A key component of the total analysis process is the 'bringing together' of findings from different sources. Part of this comes through testing the findings from one source against the findings from another. The workshops can also play a role in this. Findings are open to interpretation and the workshops can play a role in testing initial interpretation with a wider audience.

Ethics and local research governance

Evaluations come under the auspices of the Local Research Ethics Committee (LREC). It is best to seek advice from the LREC secretary or local research governance lead as to whether a particular evaluation, or any elements of it, will require approval. Guidance can also be found on the Central Office for Research Ethics Committees (COREC) website (at www.corec.org.uk). LRECs follow standard procedures and application forms are available on this website. It is almost certain that elements of the evaluation involving direct contact with service users will require formal approval by the LREC and this will require full informed and written consent. This may also apply to contact with NHS staff (via focus groups and interviews). It will also be a requirement that data is anonymised and that un-anonymised data be safeguarded. Additionally the LREC will require assurances that reporting the evaluation does not reveal the identity of subjects.

Usually the first step is to make contact with the local research governance lead, who will advise on any additional procedures the evaluation may need to go through to satisfy research governance policies, and who should also be able to advise you on approaching the LREC and their submission deadlines.

By Graham Durcan
Deputy Director of Service Development &
Criminal Justice and Mental Health Programme Lead
The Sainsbury Centre for Mental Health

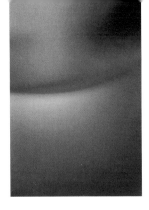

References and further reading

NOTE: Some of the unpublished audits on the Ipswich intermediate care team are available from the Sainsbury Centre for Mental Health website www.scmh.org.uk. These represent the work done as the Intermediate Care Collaborative developed, and are presented as an example of what one intermediate care team has achieved.

Abbas, A. (2005) Somatisation: diagnosing it sooner through emotion-focused interviewing. *The Journal of Family Practice*, **54** (3) 215-224.

Aziz, F., McCrone, P., Boyle, S. & Knapp, M. (2003) *Financing Mental Health Services in London.* London: King's Fund.

Barsky, A.J., Ettner, S.L., Horsky, J. & Bates, D.W. (2001) Resource utilisation of patients with hypochondriachal health anxiety and somatisation. *Med Care*, **39**, 705-15.

Bass, C. (2003) Somatisation and medically unexplained symptoms. *Psychiatry*, 1 January 2003, 15-19.

Bass, C. (ed.) (2003) Somatisation and somatoform disorders. *Psychiatry*, **2**, 10 October 2003.

Bebbington, P. (1990) Population Surveys of Psychiatric Disorder and the Need for Treatment. *Social Psychiatry and Psychiatric Epidemiology*, **25**, 33-40.

Bolton, J. (2003) What is Liaison Psychiatry? *Psychiatry*, 1 January 2003, 1-4.

Cooper, B. & Singh, B. (2000) Population Research and Mental Health Policy: Bridging the Gap. *British Journal of Psychiatry*, **176**, 407-411.

Department for Work and Pensions (2002) *Pathways to Work.* London: DWP.

Department of Health (1999) *The National Service Framework for Mental Health; Modern Standards and service models for mental health.* London: DH.

Department of Health (2000) *The NHS Plan: a plan for investment, a plan for reform.* London: DH.

Department of Health (2005) *Supporting People with Long Term Conditions: An NHS and Social Care Model to support local innovation and integration.* London: DH.

Gray, P. (1999) *Mental Health in the Workplace.* London: Mental Health Foundation.

Goldberg, D. & Huxley, P. (1992) *Common mental disorders.* Oxford: Routledge.

Hague, J. (2004) *The impact of mental illness on health services.* Unpublished. Available from: http://www.scmh.org.uk/icc [Accessed 27 September 2005].

Hague, J. (2005) *Preliminary analysis of one practices referrals to PIMHS in Ipswich.* Unpublished. Available from: http://www.scmh.org.uk/icc [Accessed 27 September 2005].

Henshall, L. (2003) *An audit of patients suitable for intermediate care.* Unpublished.

Kessler, D., Lloyd, K., Lewis, G. & Gray D.P. (1999) Cross sectional study of symptom attribution and recognition of depression and anxiety in primary care. *British Medical Journal*, **3** (318) 436-40.

Layard, R. (2004) *Mental Health: Britain's biggest social problem?* Available from: http://www.strategy.gov.uk/downloads/files/mh_layard.pdf [Accessed 27 September 2005].

Layard, R. (2005) *Therapy for all on the NHS.* Sainsbury Centre for Mental Health Lecture. 12 September 2005. Available from: http://www.scmh.org.uk

Little, M. (2003) *Audit of acute assessment team referrals in Ipswich.* Unpublished.

Murray, C.J.L. & Lopez, A.D. (1996) *The global burden of disease.* Boston, Mass: WHO and Harvard University Press.

National Institute for Health and Clinical Excellence (2004a) *Depression, Management of depression in primary and secondary care.* London: NICE.

National Institute for Health and Clinical Excellence (2004b) *Anxiety, Management of anxiety in primary and secondary care.* London: NICE.

Nimnuan, M., Hotopf, M. & Wesseley, S. (2000) Medically unexplained symptoms, how often and why are they missed? *QJMed,* **93**, 21-28.

Office for National Statistics (2000) *Psychiatric Morbidity Among Adults Living in Private Households.* Technical Report. London: HMSO.

Ranzetta, T. (2005) *The economic benefit of an Intermediate Care Team in Ipswich.* Unpublished.

Reid, S., Wesseley, S., Vrayford, T. & Hotopf, M. (2002) Frequent attenders with medically unexplained symptoms: service use and costs in secondary care. *British Journal of Psychiatry,* **180**, 248-253.

Roberts, M. (2004) *An audit of referrals to East Ipswich CMHT.* Unpublished. Available from: http://www.scmh.org.uk/icc [Accessed 27 September 2005].

Robson, C. (2002) *Real World Research: A resource for social scientists and practitioner-researchers.* 2nd edition. London: Blackwell.

Rost, K., Nutting, P., Smith, J.L., Elliott, C.E. & Dickinson, M. (2002) Managing depression as a chronic disease: a randomised trial of ongoing treatment in primary care. *British Medical Journal,* **325**, 934.

The Sainsbury Centre for Mental Health (2000) *Taking Your Partners: Using opportunities for inter-agency partnership in mental health.* London: SCMH.

The Sainsbury Centre for Mental Health (2002) *Primary Solutions: An independent policy review on the development of primary care mental health services.* London: SCMH.

The Sainsbury Centre for Mental Health (2003) *The economic and social costs of mental illness. Policy Paper 3.* London: SCMH.

Social Exclusion Unit (2004) *Mental Health and Social Exclusion: Social Exclusion Unit Report.* London: Office of the Deputy Prime Minister.

World Health Organisation – UK Collaborating Centre (2004) *WHO guide to Mental and Neurological Health in Primary Care.* WHO: London. Available from: http://www.mentalneurologicalprimarycare.org [Accessed 27 September 2005].